58 Stroke Preventive Meal Recipes:

The Stroke-Survivors Solution to a Healthy Diet and Long Life

By

Joe Correa CSN

COPYRIGHT

This publication is designed to provide accurate and authoritative information in regard to the subject matter covered. It is sold with the understanding that neither the author nor the publisher is engaged in rendering medical advice. If medical advice or assistance is needed, consult with a doctor. This book is considered a guide and should not be used in any way detrimental to your health. Consult with a physician before starting this nutritional plan to make sure it's right for you.

ACKNOWLEDGEMENTS

This book is dedicated to my friends and family that have had mild or serious illnesses so that you may find a solution and make the necessary changes in your life.

58 Stroke Preventive Meal Recipes:

The Stroke-Survivors Solution to a Healthy Diet and Long Life

By

Joe Correa CSN

CONTENTS

ABOUT THE AUTHOR

After years of Research, I honestly believe in the positive effects that proper nutrition can have over the body and mind. My knowledge and experience has helped me live healthier throughout the years and which I have shared with family and friends. The more you know about eating and drinking healthier, the sooner you will want to change your life and eating habits.

Nutrition is a key part in the process of being healthy and living longer so get started today. The first step is the most important and the most significant.

INTRODUCTION

58 Stroke Preventive Meal Recipes: The Stroke-Survivors Solution to a Healthy Diet and Long Life

By Joe Correa CSN

Stroke is one of the main causes of death in the world. Modern lifestyles, poor diets, and sedentary jobs are the underlying cause of some surprising statistics. In the USA about 800,000 people die due to stroke each year. Along with heart disease, cancer, and accidents, stroke is the leading cause of death and should be taken seriously.

Bearing in mind that every 40 seconds someone dies from a stroke, it is important to start thinking about the entire cardiovascular system and its health, including the heart. Prevention is a key to reducing the possibility of this terrible disease.

A stroke happens when the blood supply to the brain is interrupted. This can happen when the entire blood vessel is blocked or the brain blood vessel is ruptured. In both cases, it causes the brain tissue to die, leading to quick and sudden death. This is exactly why a stroke is a serious medical condition and should be treated as quick as possible.

However, you have to keep in mind that a stroke can easily be prevented. The main problem lies in bad nutritional habits that should be replaced with good and healthy eating habits. This primarily includes fresh, raw, organic, and healthy foods that will help your body to deal with daily challenges and heal itself at the same time.

This book is an excellent collection of recipes that will help your cardiovascular system to function better than ever and reduce the risk of having a stroke. These recipes are based on organic and natural foods that are full of healthy fats, carbs, proteins, vitamins, and minerals.

Besides, this book offers some amazingly delicious solutions and ways of preparing these dishes. Numerous combinations will quickly replace your usual breakfast, lunch, snack, or even typical dinner recipes. Try every single one of them to which one you like the most and enjoy a healthy life!

58 STROKE PREVENTIVE MEAL RECIPES: THE STROKE-SURVIVORS SOLUTION TO A HEALTHY DIET AND LONG LIFE

1.   Sweet Potato Frittata

Ingredients:

6 large eggs, beaten

1 medium-sized bell pepper, sliced

1 small red onion, finely chopped

1 cup of sweet potatoes, cubed

2 garlic cloves, crushed

¼ cup of Cheddar cheese, grated

1 tbsp of fresh parsley, finely chopped

1 tbsp of extra-virgin olive oil

Preparation:

First, you need to prepare the vegetables. Place the potatoes in a pot of boiling water and cook for 10 minutes, or until fork-tender. Remove from the heat and drain well. Set aside.

Whisk in the eggs, parsley, and cheese in a medium bowl. Mix until well incorporated and set aside.

Now, preheat the oil in a large nonstick frying pan over a medium-high temperature. Add crushed garlic, onion, and pepper and cook for 3-4 minutes, stirring occasionally.

Add the potatoes and cook for another 3 minutes. pour the egg mixture over the vegetables and stir to spread evenly. Cook until eggs are set and remove from the heat.

Serve immediately.

Nutritional information per serving: Kcal: 229, Protein: 12.4g, Carbs: 15.6g, Fats: 13g

2.   Potato with Garlic

Ingredients:

3 large potatoes, peeled and wedged

3 tbsp of extra-virgin olive oil

4 garlic cloves, minced

1 small onion, finely chopped

1 tbsp of fresh thyme, finely chopped

1 tsp of fresh rosemary, finely chopped

¼ tsp of black pepper, freshly ground

Preparation:

Place the potatoes in a pot of boiling water and cook for 10 minutes, or until tender. Remove from the heat and drain well. Refresh under cold running water and then drain again. Set aside.

Preheat the oil in a small saucepan over a medium-high temperature. Add garlic and onion and cook for 3 minutes. Stir in the thyme, rosemary, and pepper. Cook for 2 minutes more and remove from the heat.

Preheat the grill to a medium-high temperature. Brush the potatoes with oil mixture and grill for 8-10 minutes, or until slightly browned.

Transfer the potatoes to a serving plate and drizzle with the remaining mixture. Top with sour cream and serve immediately.

Nutritional information per serving: Kcal: 383, Protein: 6.1g, Carbs: 48g, Fats: 19.8g

3.   Veal and Peppers in Milk Sauce

Ingredients:

1 lb of lean veal, cut into bite-sized pieces

½ cup of chicken stock, unsalted

2 large red bell peppers, seeded and halved

4 tbsp of milk, low-fat

1 small onion, finely chopped

1 tbsp of olive oil

¼ tsp of black pepper, ground

Preparation:

Preheat the oil in a large saucepan over a medium-high temperature. Add meat chops and cook for 5 minutes, stirring occasionally. Pour the chicken stock and cook for another 5 minutes, until almost all the liquid evaporates. Remove the meat and reserve the saucepan.

Throw in the garlic and onion. Cook until translucent and then add pepper halves. Cook for 2-3 minutes, or until peppers slightly soften. Pour in the milk and cook for 2 minutes. Remove from the heat.

Serve meat with peppers and drizzle with the remaining milk sauce from the saucepan. Serve warm.

Nutritional information per serving: Kcal: 260, Protein: 29g, Carbs: 7g, Fats: 12.6g

4.   Orange Peach Smoothie

Ingredients:

2 large peaches, pitted and chopped

1 large orange, peeled

1 cup of milk, low-fat

½ tsp of cherry extract

1 large banana

1 tbsp of sunflower seeds

Preparation:

Wash the peaches and cut in half. Remove the pits and cut into small pieces. Transfer to a food processor.

Peel the orange and divide into wedges. Transfer to a food processor. Peel the banana and cut into chunks. Transfer to a food processor along with milk, cherry extract, and banana. Blend for 2 minutes or until smooth and creamy.

Transfer to serving glasses and top with sunflower seeds. Refrigerate for 15 minutes before serving.

Enjoy!

Nutritional information per serving: Kcal: 157, Protein: 4.9g, Carbs: 31.2g, Fats: 2.6g

5.   Scrambled Eggs with Mushrooms

Ingredients:

1 cup of button mushrooms, sliced

1 large green bell pepper, sliced

5 large eggs

1 tbsp of scallions

½ tsp of dried oregano, ground

2 tbsp of milk, low-fat

1 tbsp of olive oil

¼ tsp of black pepper, ground

Preparation:

Preheat the oil in a large nonstick skillet over a medium-high temperature. Add mushrooms and bell pepper. Cook for 5 minutes, or until slightly tender. Stir occasionally.

Meanwhile, whisk the eggs with scallions, oregano, milk, and pepper. Pour the mixture into a skillet and fry for 3-5 minutes. Using a wooden spatula, scrape out the eggs from the bottom of the skillet to cook evenly.

Remove from the heat and serve immediately.

Nutritional information per serving: Kcal: 276, Protein: 18.1g, Carbs: 8g, Fats: 20.1g

6.　　Warm Carrot Oatmeal

Ingredients:

1 cup of rolled oats

1 cup of milk, low-fat

1 cup of carrots, pre-cooked

¼ tsp of cinnamon, ground

1 tbsp of flaxseeds

1 tbsp of honey

1 tbsp of Brazil nuts, roughly chopped

Preparation:

Wash and peel the carrots. Chop into thin slices and place in a pot of boiling water. Cook for 15 minutes, or until soften. Remove from the heat and drain. Set aside to cool for a while.

Meanwhile, combine oats, milk, cinnamon, and honey in a fire-proof dish. Place it in a microwave for 3 minutes and set aside.

Now, place the carrots in a food processor or a blender. Process until pureed and add it to the oats. Stir all well and reheat in a microwave to the desired temperature.

Sprinkle with nuts and flaxseeds before serving.

Enjoy!

Nutritional information per serving: Kcal: 322, Protein: 11.2g, Carbs: 49.6g, Fats: 9.6g

7.   Trout with Pasta

Ingredients:

1 lb of trout fillets

8 oz of pasta

1 cup of tomato sauce

2 tbsp of extra-virgin olive oil

1 tbsp of balsamic vinegar

2 garlic cloves, minced

1 tsp of Italian seasoning mix

¼ tsp of dried oregano, ground

1 tbsp of fresh parsley, finely chopped

1 tbsp of lemon juice, freshly squeezed

Preparation:

Prepare the pasta using package instructions. Drain the pasta and set aside.

Preheat the oil in a large skillet over a medium-high temperature. Add garlic and saute for 2-3 minutes, or until translucent. Now, add fish fillets and sprinkle with balsamic vinegar, Italian seasoning mix, oregano, and lemon juice. Cook the fillets for 5 minutes on both sides, or until set. Remove from the heat.

Now, transfer pasta to serving plates and top with fish fillets. Sprinkle with parsley and serve immediately.

Nutritional information per serving: Kcal: 458, Protein: 37.6g, Carbs: 35.1g, Fats: 18.1g

8.   Strawberry Spinach Salad

Ingredients:

10 oz of fresh spinach, roughly chopped

1 cup of strawberries, chopped

1 medium-sized cucumber, sliced

2 tbsp of almonds, roughly chopped

2 tbsp of orange juice, freshly juiced

1 tbsp of extra-virgin olive oil

1 tbsp of honey

Preparation:

Combine almonds, orange juice, oil, and honey in a medium bowl. Stir well and set aside.

Wash the spinach thoroughly under cold running water. Drain and roughly chop it. Set aside.

Wash the strawberries and cut into bite-sized pieces. Set aside.

Wash the cucumber and chop it into thin slices. Set aside.

Now, combine spinach, strawberries, and cucumber in a salad bowl. Stir well and then drizzle with previously prepared sauce. Toss well to coat and refrigerate for 20 minutes before serving.

Enjoy!

Nutritional information per serving: Kcal: 141, Protein: 4.6g, Carbs: 18.4g, Fats: 7.3g

9.   Kidney Beans Stew

Ingredients:

10 oz of kidney beans, soaked overnight

1 cup of canned tomatoes, diced

1 tbsp of tomato paste

1 medium-sized bell pepper

1 tbsp of olive oil

1 small onion, finely chopped

2 garlic cloves, crushed

1 medium-sized potato, chopped

2 cups of water

Preparation:

Soak the beans overnight. Drain well and rinse under cold running water. Drain again and set aside.

Place the beans in a deep pot and add 3 cups of water. Bring it to a boil and continue to cook for 15 minutes. Remove from the heat, drain, and set aside.

Peel the potato and cut into small chunks. Place it in a pot of boiling water and cook for 5 minutes. Remove from the heat and drain well. Set aside.

Preheat the oil in a heavy-bottomed pot over a medium-high temperature. Add garlic and onions and stir-fry for 3-4 minutes, or until translucent.

Now, add all other ingredients and bring it to a boil. Reduce the heat to low and cover with a lid. Cook for 30 minutes and remove from the heat.

Serve warm.

Nutritional information per serving: Kcal: 227, Protein: 12.1g, Carbs: 39.8g, Fats: 3g

10.   Tuna Steaks with Cherry Tomatoes

Ingredients:

2 lbs of tuna steaks

3 garlic cloves, crushed

4 tbsp of extra-virgin olive oil

1 tsp of fresh coriander, finely chopped

1 tbsp of fresh rosemary, finely chopped

2 tbsp of lemon juice, freshly squeezed

¼ tsp of black pepper, freshly ground

1 cup of cherry tomatoes, halved

Preparation:

Wash the tuna steaks under cold running water and pat dry with a kitchen paper.

In a small bowl, combine oil, garlic, coriander, rosemary, lemon juice, and pepper. Stir well until well incorporated. Spread this mixture over the tuna steaks.

Preheat the grill to a medium-high temperature. Grill the steaks for about 5-7 minutes on both sides, or until desired doneness. Serve steaks with fresh cherry tomatoes.

Nutritional information per serving: Kcal: 369, Protein: 45.7g, Carbs: 2.2g, Fats: 19g

11.   Creamy Blackberry Salad

Ingredients:

1 cup of fresh blackberries

1 cup of strawberries, halved

1 large Granny Smith's apple, cut into bite-sized pieces

1 large cucumber, sliced

1 cup of sour cream, low-fat

1 tbsp of honey, raw

2 tbsp of olive oil

2 tbsp of almonds, roughly chopped

1 tbsp of walnuts, roughly chopped

Preparation:

Wash and prepare the fruits and vegetables.

Combine sour cream, almonds, walnuts, honey, and oil in a medium bowl. Set aside to allow flavors to meld.

Now, combine blackberries, strawberries, apple, and cucumber in a large salad bowl. Add sour cream mixture and stir well to coat all the ingredients.

Refrigerate for 15 minutes before serving and enjoy!

Nutritional information per serving: Kcal: 296, Protein: 4.3g, Carbs: 24.3g, Fats: 22.2g

12.   Grilled Salmon with Potatoes

Ingredients:

2 lbs of salmon fillets

2 large potatoes, cut into bite-sized pieces

3 tbsp of lemon juice, freshly squeezed

3 garlic cloves, crushed

1 tbsp of fresh basil, finely chopped

1 tbsp of fresh rosemary, finely chopped

4 tbsp of olive oil

¼ tsp of black pepper, ground

Preparation:

Wash the fillets under cold running water and pat dry with a kitchen paper. Set aside.

Peel the potatoes and cut into bite-sized pieces. Place the potatoes in a pot of boiling water and cook for 15 minutes, or until fork-tender. Remove from the heat and drain. Set aside.

In a large bowl, combine olive oil, garlic, rosemary, basil, lemon juice, and pepper. Stir well to combine and set aside.

Preheat the grill to a medium-high temperature. Gently brush the fillets with sauce and place on a grill.

Grill for 2-3 minutes on each side, or until doneness. Remove from the heat and transfer to a serving plate. Add potatoes and drizzle with the remaining sauce. Serve immediately.

Nutritional information per serving: Kcal: 388, Protein: 31.6g, Carbs: 20.4g, Fats: 20.9g

13.   Creamy Leek Soup

Ingredients:

1 cup of leeks, chopped

1 medium-sized potato

1 large carrot, chopped

1 cup of chicken stock, unsalted

1 cup of milk, low-fat

1 cup of spinach, finely chopped

1 tbsp of parsley, finely chopped

¼ tsp of black pepper, ground

Preparation:

Wash and prepare the vegetables. Place the leeks, spinach, and celery in a pot of boiling water. Cook for 3 minutes and remove from the heat. Drain well and set aside.

Place the potato in a pot of boiling water and cook for 5 minutes, or until slightly tender. Remove from the heat and drain well. Set aside.

Now, combine leeks, potato, carrot, and spinach in a heavy-bottomed pot. Pour the chicken stock and milk. Sprinkle with pepper and parsley. Bring it to a boil and then reduce the heat to low. Simmer for 15 minutes and remove from the heat.

Serve warm.

Nutritional information per serving: Kcal: 89, Protein: 4g, Carbs: 17.8g, Fats: 0.3g

14.   Banana Almond Smoothie

Ingredients:

1 large banana, chopped

2 tbsp of almonds

1 cup of Greek yogurt

1 small carrot, sliced

1 tsp of vanilla extract

Preparation:

Peel the banana and chop into small chunks. Set aside.

Peel the carrots and cut into thin slices. Set aside.

Now, combine banana, carrots, almonds, yogurt, and vanilla extract in a food processor or a blender. Blend until nicely smooth and transfer to serving glasses. Sprinkle with some extra almonds and add some ice before serving.

Enjoy!

Nutritional information per serving: Kcal: 202, Protein: 14.3g, Carbs: 24.4g, Fats: 5.6g

15.   Shiitake Collard Greens

Ingredients:

1 cup of Shiitake mushrooms, chopped

2 cups of collard greens, chopped

2 garlic cloves, minced

2 tbsp of extra-virgin olive oil

2 tbsp of lemon juice, freshly squeezed

1 tbsp of Dijon mustard

¼ tsp of black pepper

½ cup of chicken broth, unsalted

Preparation:

In a medium bowl, combine 1 tablespoon of olive oil, garlic, lemon juice, mustard, and pepper. Stir until well incorporated and set aside.

Preheat the remaining oil in a large nonstick saucepan over a medium-high temperature. Add mushrooms and cook for 10 minutes. Transfer mushrooms to a bowl and reserve the pan.

Pour the chicken broth into the pan and add garlic. Bring it to a boil and then add collard greens. Cook for 5 minutes then reduce the heat. Add mushrooms and cook for another 2 minutes. Remove from the heat and transfer to a serving plate. Drizzle with previously made sauce and serve immediately.

Nutritional information per serving: Kcal: 185, Protein: 4g, Carbs: 14.5g, Fats: 14g

16.   Turkey Breasts with Zucchini

Ingredients:

1 lb of turkey breasts, skinless and boneless

1 large zucchini, peeled and chopped

3 garlic cloves, minced

1 small onion, finely chopped

3 tbsp of extra-virgin olive oil

¼ tsp of black pepper, ground

Preparation:

Peel the zucchinis and cut in half. Scrape out the seeds and chop into small chunks. Place in a pot of boiling water and cook for 5 minutes, or until tender. Set aside.

Now, preheat the oil in a large frying pan over a medium-high temperature. Add garlic and onions and cook for 3 minutes, or until translucent. Add turkey breasts and cook for 10 minutes more, stirring occasionally. Throw in the zucchinis and sprinkle with some pepper. Cook for 3 minutes more and remove from the heat.

Serve immediately.

Nutritional information per serving: Kcal: 232, Protein: 20.7g, Carbs: 9.9g, Fats: 12.6g

17.   Lean Shrimp Stew with Brussels Sprouts

Ingredients:

1 lb of large shrimps, cleaned and deveined

7 oz of Brussels sprouts, trimmed

5 oz of okra

2 small carrots, sliced

3 oz of baby corn

2 cups of chicken broth

2 large tomatoes, diced

2 tbsp of tomato paste

½ tsp of chili pepper, ground

¼ tsp of black pepper, freshly ground

½ cup of olive oil

1 tbsp of balsamic vinegar

1 tbsp of fresh rosemary, finely chopped

1 small celery stalk, for decoration

2 tbsp of sour cream

Preparation:

Wash the shrimps under cold running water and pat dry with a kitchen paper. Set aside.

Combine 3 tablespoons of olive oil, balsamic vinegar, rosemary, and pepper in a large bowl. Stir well and place the shrimps into the bowl. Toss well to coat and refrigerate for 20 minutes to allow flavors to meld into the shrimps.

Meanwhile, wash and prepare the vegetables. Trim off the outer layers of the Brussels sprouts and slice the carrots.

Now, preheat the remaining oil in a heavy-bottomed pot over a medium-high temperature. Add Brussels sprouts, okra, carrots and celery. Saute for 5 minutes. Add tomatoes, tomato paste, and chili. Sprinkle with some pepper and stir well to combine. Cook for 3 minutes more.

Drain the shrimps and add to the pot. Pour about 2 cups of water and give it a good stir. Reduce the heat to low and cook for 15 minutes. Add corn and cook for 3 minutes more. Remove from the heat and transfer to a serving plate. Top with sour cream and drizzle little bit with a shrimp marinade.

Nutrition information per serving: Kcal: 193, Protein: 15.7g, Carbs: 20.1g, Fats: 7.2g

18.   Sweet Potato Tuna

Ingredients:

1 lb of tuna fillets

4 tbsp of olive oil

1 tbsp of balsamic vinegar

2 tbsp of lemon juice

1 tbsp of toasted almonds

¼ tsp of black pepper, ground

1 medium-sized sweet potato

Preparation:

In a medium bowl, combine oil, vinegar, lemon juice, almond, and pepper. Mix well and set aside to allow flavors to blend.

Peel the potato and cut into small chunks. Place it in a pot of boiling water. Cook for 20 minutes, or until fork-tender. Remove from the heat and set aside.

Preheat the electric grill to a medium-high temperature. Brush the tuna fillets with marinade and grill for about 2-3 minutes on each side.

Transfer to a serving plate and serve with potatoes. Drizzle all with marinade and serve immediately.

Nutrition information per serving: Kcal: 491, Protein: 41.4g, Carbs: 8.7g, Fats: 32g

19.   Pineapple Salad

Ingredients:

1 cup of pineapple chunks

1 large mango, chopped

1 cup of Iceberg lettuce, torn

1 cup of fresh spinach, torn

1 cup of blueberries

4 tbsp of orange juice, freshly juiced

2 tbsp of lemon juice

1 tbsp of honey

2 tbsp of walnuts, roughly chopped

Preparation:

Combine orange juice, lemon juice, honey, and walnuts in a small bowl. Mix until well incorporated and set aside to allow flavors to mingle. Set aside.

Wash and prepare the fruits and vegetables.

Peel and cut the pineapple and mango into small chunks and set aside.

In a large colander, combine lettuce and spinach and wash under cold running water. Torn with hands and set aside.

Wash the blueberries and combine along with pineapple, mango, lettuce, and spinach in a large salad bowl. Drizzle with marinade and refrigerate for 15 minutes before serving.

Enjoy!

Nutrition information per serving: Kcal: 192, Protein: 3.5g, Carbs: 40.5g, Fats: 3.9g

20.   Creamy Quinoa with Dates

Ingredients:

1 cup of quinoa, pre-cooked

¼ cup of dates, chopped

1 tbsp of cashews, roughly chopped

1 tsp of pumpkin seeds

¼ tsp of cinnamon, ground

1 cup of milk, low-fat

1 tbsp of honey

Preparation:

Place the quinoa in a deep pot. Add 3 cups of water and bring it to a boil. Reduce the heat to low and cook for 15 minutes. Remove from the heat and drain. Stir once and set aside.

Now, combine quinoa, dates, cinnamon, cashews, milk, and honey in a medium bowl. Stir well to combine and transfer to serving dishes.

Top with pumpkin seeds and serve immediately.

Nutrition information per serving: Kcal: 192, Protein: 3.5g, Carbs: 40.5g, Fats: 3.9g

21.   Cherry Muffins

Ingredients:

2 cups of buckwheat flour

7 oz of cherries, pitted

3 tsp of baking powder

1 cup of milk, low-fat

6 tbsp of cream cheese, low-fat

1 tbsp of liquid honey

2 large eggs

1 large pear, peeled, cored, and finely chopped

Preparation:

Preheat the oven to 400°F.

In a medium bowl, combine flour and baking powder. Stir well and set aside.

Wash the cherries and pear. Cut the cherries in half and remove the pits. Peel the pear and remove the core. Cut into bite-sized pieces and set aside.

Now, combine pear, cherries, eggs, milk, and honey in a large bowl. Stir well to combine and pour this mixture over a flour mixture. Stir well until you get nice dough.

Grease muffin molds with some oil and spoon the mixture evenly. Top with each muffin with cream cheese.

Place it in the oven and bake for 25 minutes, or until set. Remove from the oven and set aside to cool.

Serve warm.

Nutritional information per serving: Kcal: 278, Protein: 9.4g, Carbs: 47.5g, Fats: 7.3g

22.   Strawberry Banana Smoothie

Ingredients:

1 cup of strawberries

1 large banana

1 cup of milk, low-fat

1 tbsp pumpkin seeds

1 tsp of vanilla extract

Preparation:

Wash the strawberries under cold running water and cut in half. transfer to a food processor.

Peel the banana and cut into chunks. Add it to the food processor along with milk and vanilla extract. Blend for 2 minutes or until smooth and creamy.

Transfer to serving glasses and top with pumpkin seeds. Refrigerate for 15 minutes, or add some ice before serving.

Enjoy!

Nutritional information per serving: Kcal: 116, Protein: 4.2g, Carbs: 18.7g, Fats: 3.3g

23. Celery Nutmeg Omelet

Ingredients:

1 cup of celery, finely chopped

1 large red onion, chopped

¼ tsp of nutmeg, ground

6 large eggs

1 tbsp of milk, low-fat

1 tbsp of olive oil

Preparation:

In a medium bowl, whisk together eggs with nutmeg, and milk. Set aside.

Wash and prepare the celery and onion. Set aside.

Preheat the oil in a large nonstick frying pan over a medium-high temperature. Add onion and stir-fry for 2 minutes. Now, add celery and continue to cook for 2 more minutes.

Pour the egg mixture into the pan and cook for 3-4 minutes, or until eggs are set. Fold the omelet and remove from the pan.

Serve immediately.

Nutritional information per serving: Kcal: 212, Protein: 13.5g, Carbs: 6.8g, Fats: 14.9g

24.   Creamy Leek Artichoke Soup

Ingredients:

1 lb of leeks, chopped

1 medium-sized onion

1 cup of artichoke, chopped

1 tbsp of olive oil

1 tbsp of fresh parsley, finely chopped

3 cups of vegetable broth, unsalted

2 tbsp of lemon juice, freshly squeezed

¼ tsp of black pepper, ground

Preparation:

Preheat the oil in a heavy-bottomed pot over a medium-high temperature. Add onions and stir-fry for about 2-3 minutes.

Now, add leeks, artichokes, and lemon juice. Stir well and cook for 2 minutes. Add vegetable broth and sprinkle with some pepper to taste. Stir again and cook for 15 minutes. Remove from the heat.

Using a large colander, drain all the liquid to another pot. Transfer the vegetables to a food processor and blend well until smooth. Return to a pot with broth. Heat it up for 4-5 minutes and serve immediately.

Nutritional information per serving: Kcal: 102, Protein: 4.5g, Carbs: 15.4g, Fats: 4.5g

25.   Baked Veal with Carrots

Ingredients:

1 lb of lean veal, cut into bite-sized pieces

1 tbsp of buckwheat flour

2 tbsp of olive oil

1 medium-sized carrot, chopped

1 cup of tomato sauce

1 tbsp of balsamic vinegar

¼ tsp of black pepper, freshly ground

1 tbsp of fresh thyme, finely chopped

Preparation:

Preheat the oven to 400°F.

Combine flour, vinegar, tomato sauce, vinegar, and one tablespoon of olive oil. Stir well until combined and set aside.

Grease a large baking sheet with oil. Spread the meat chops evenly onto it. Sprinkle with pepper, and thyme, and squeeze with your hands to rub in the spices. Tuck in the carrot slices between the meat chops and place it in the oven.

Bake for about 15 minutes and then add the tomato sauce mixture. Spread evenly and continue to bake for 5 more minutes. Remove from the oven and serve warm.

Nutritional information per serving: Kcal: 102, Protein: 4.5g, Carbs: 15.4g, Fats: 4.5g

26.   Apricot Oatmeal with Flaxseeds

Ingredients:

4 medium-sized apricots, chopped

1 cup of milk, low-fat

1 tbsp of honey

1 tbsp of flaxseeds

1 cup of oatmeal

Preparation:

Wash the apricots and cut in half. Remove the pits and cut into small pieces. Transfer to a deep pot and add 2 cups of water. Bring it to a boil and cook for 2 minutes. Remove from the heat and drain. Set aside to cool for a while.

Combine oatmeal, milk, honey, and flaxseeds. Stir well and place it in a microwave. Heat it up for 1 minute and then stir in the apricots.

Serve immediately.

Nutritional information per serving: Kcal: 300, Protein: 11g, Carbs: 51g, Fats: 6.7g

27. Turkey Breasts with Arugula Cream

Ingredients:

1 lb of turkey breasts, skinless and boneless

1 cup of fresh arugula, chopped

1 large tomato, diced

3 tbsp of olive oil

2 tbsp of lemon juice, freshly squeezed

½ tsp of black pepper, freshly ground

1 tsp of dried thyme, ground

Preparation:

In a large bowl, combine arugula, tomato, lemon juice, and pepper. Stir well to combine and transfer to a blender. Process until creamy and set aside.

Preheat the oil in a large nonstick skillet over a medium-high temperature. Add turkey breasts and sprinkle with thyme. Cook for 4-5 minutes on each side, or until desired doneness.

Transfer to a serving plate and pour over the arugula cream. Serve with some lemon wedges or sprinkle with lemon zest. However, this is optional.

Enjoy!

Nutritional information per serving: Kcal: 294, Protein: 26.7g, Carbs: 9.6g, Fats: 16.8g

28.   Sweet Potato Pasta

Ingredients:

1 lb of whole-grain penne pasta

2 large tomatoes, diced

3 tbsp of tomato paste

2 medium-sized sweet potatoes, chopped

2 tbsp of sour cream

1 tbsp of balsamic vinegar

1 tsp of dried oregano

½ tsp of Italian seasoning mix

1 tbsp of fresh parsley, finely chopped

Preparation:

Cook the pasta using package instructions. Remove from the heat and drain well. Set aside.

Peel the potatoes and chop into small pieces. Place in a pot of boiling water and cook until fork-tender. Remove from the heat and drain well. Set aside to cool for a while.

Preheat the oil in a large skillet over a medium-high temperature. Add tomatoes, tomato paste, oregano, and Italian seasoning mix. Stir well and cook for 2 minutes. Add sweet potatoes and sour cream. Cook for 2 minutes more and remove from the heat.

Transfer the pasta to serving plates and top with tomato sauce. Sprinkle with some fresh parsley and serve immediately.

Nutritional information per serving: Kcal: 304, Protein: 10.4g, Carbs: 59.6g, Fats: 2.9g

29. Bell Pepper Polenta

Ingredients:

1 cup of cornstarch

3 cups of water

1 small onion, finely chopped

1 medium-sized red bell pepper, chopped

1 medium-sized green bell pepper, chopped

1 tbsp of vegetable oil

½ cup of sour cream, low-fat

Preparation:

Pour the water in a deep pot. Bring it to a boil and then gently stir in the cornstarch. Cook for 20 minutes on medium temperature. Stir constantly until mixture nicely thickens. Remove from the heat and set aside.

Preheat the oil in a medium nonstick skillet over a medium-high temperature. Add onion and stir-fry until translucent. Now, add peppers and cook for 5 minutes, or until peppers soften. Remove from the heat and set aside.

Transfer the polenta to serving plates and spoon the peppers and onion. Top with sour cream and serve immediately.

Nutritional information per serving: Kcal: 304, Protein: 10.4g, Carbs: 59.6g, Fats: 2.9g

30.   Green Bean Brussels Sprout Stew

Ingredients:

1 cup of green beans, chopped

1 cup of Brussel sprouts, chopped

2 cups of vegetable broth

1 large carrot, chopped

1 cup of sweet potatoes, chopped

1 large tomato, diced

2 tbsp of tomato paste

1 tsp of cayenne pepper, ground

¼ tsp of black pepper, ground

2 tbsp of olive oil

1 tsp of dried thyme, ground

Preparation:

Place the sweet potatoes in a pot of boiling water. Cook for 10 minutes and then remove from the heat. Drain and set aside.

Preheat the oil in a heavy-bottomed pot over a medium-high temperature. Add Brussels sprouts, carrots, and green beans. Cook for 5 minutes, stirring occasionally. Now, pour the broth and add tomato. Stir and cook for 10 minutes. Reduce the heat to low.

Stir in the tomato paste and sprinkle with pepper, cayenne pepper, and thyme.

Cook for 5 minutes more and remove from the heat.

Enjoy!

Nutritional information per serving: Kcal: 133, Protein: 4.2g, Carbs: 16.3g, Fats: 6.5g

58 Stroke Preventive Meal Recipes

31.   Trout with Potato Puree

Ingredients:

1 lb of trout fillets

1 cup of sweet potatoes, chopped

½ cup of spring onions, finely chopped

3 tbsp of olive oil

2 tbsp of lemon juice, freshly squeezed

3 garlic cloves, crushed

½ tsp of black pepper, ground

1 tbsp of fresh rosemary, finely chopped

1 tsp of balsamic vinegar

Preparation:

Place chopped potatoes in a pot of boiling water and cook for 10 minutes. Remove from the heat and drain well. Set aside.

In a small bowl, combine olive oil, lemon juice, garlic, pepper, and rosemary. Stir well to combine and set aside.

Preheat the grill to a medium-high temperature. Brush the fillets with marinade and grill for 3-4 minutes on each side. Brush occasionally when dried out. Transfer the fillets to a bowl and cover with a lid. Set aside.

Now, place the potatoes and remaining marinade into a food processor. Blend until smooth and set aside.

Serve the fillets with potato puree.

Nutritional information per serving: Kcal: 363, Protein: 31.3g, Carbs: 13g, Fats: 20.4g

32.   Watermelon Kale Smoothie

Ingredients:

1 cup of fresh kale, chopped

1 cup of watermelon chunks

1 tsp of turmeric, ground

1 tbsp of liquid honey

½ cup of sour cream, low-fat

Preparation:

Wash the kale thoroughly under cold running water. Drain and roughly chop it. Set aside.

Peel the watermelon lengthwise in half. Cut one large wedge and peel it. Chop into chunks and discard the seeds. Set aside.

Now, combine kale, watermelon, turmeric, honey, and sour cream in a food processor or a blender. Process until smooth and creamy. Transfer to serving glasses and refrigerate for 15 minutes before serving.

Enjoy!

Nutritional information per serving: Kcal: 198, Protein: 3.4g, Carbs: 21g, Fats: 12.3g

33. Kiwi Raspberry Salad

Ingredients:

2 large kiwis, chopped

1 cup of raspberries

1 cup of watermelon, chopped

1 large peach, chopped

2 tbsp of lemon juice, freshly squeezed

2 tbsp of orange juice, freshly squeezed

2 tbsp of walnuts, roughly chopped

Preparation:

In a small bowl, combine lemon juice, orange juice, and walnuts. Stir and set aside.

Wash the peach and cut in half. Remove the pit and cut into bite-sized pieces. Wash the raspberries under cold running water. Peel the kiwis and cut lengthwise in half.

Cut the watermelon in half. Cut one large wedge and peel it. Discard the seeds and fill the measuring cup. Wrap the rest in a plastic foil and refrigerate.

Now, combine kiwis, raspberries, watermelon, and peach in a large salad bowl. Drizzle with the dressing and toss well to combine all the ingredients.

Refrigerate for 15 minutes before serving.

Nutritional information per serving: Kcal: 126, Protein: 3.2g, Carbs: 22.6g, Fats: 3.9g

34.   Chicken with Brown Rice

Ingredients:

1 lb of chicken breasts, skinless and boneless

1 cup of brown rice

¼ cup of spring onions, finely chopped

1 small carrot, sliced

2 tbsp of olive oil

¼ tsp of turmeric, ground

¼ tsp of black pepper, ground

¼ tsp of dried oregano, ground

Preparation:

Place the rice in a heavy-bottomed pot. Add 3 cups of water and bring it to a boil. Cook for 15 minutes, then reduce the heat to low. Stir in the turmeric and cook for 2 minutes more. Remove from the heat. Stir in the green onions and set aside.

Preheat the oil in a large skillet over a medium-high temperature. Add onions and carrot and cook for 3-4 minutes.

Now, add meat and sprinkle with some pepper, and oregano. Cook for about 4-5 minutes or until desired doneness. Remove from the heat and transfer to a serving plate.

Serve the chicken breasts with rice and enjoy.

Nutritional information per serving: Kcal: 456, Protein: 36.6g, Carbs: 38.1g, Fats: 16.7g

35.   Green Muffins

Ingredients:

2 cups of buckwheat flour

¼ cup of spinach

1 tbsp of sour cream, low-fat

1 tbsp of baking powder

1 cup of milk, low-fat

2 large eggs

Preparation:

Preheat the oven to 300°F.

In a large bowl, combine flour and baking powder. Set aside.

In a separate bowl, combine eggs, sour cream, and milk. Whisk well and set aside.

Using a hand electric mixer, gently stir in the egg mixture into flour mixture. Finally, add spinach and mix until you get the nice smooth dough.

Spoon the muffins into muffin molds. Place it in the oven and bake for about 20-25 minutes, or until set.

Serve warm.

Nutritional information per serving: Kcal: 185, Protein: 8.6g, Carbs: 31.7g, Fats: 4.2g

36.   Tomato Eggplant Stew

Ingredients:

2 large tomatoes, peeled and diced

1 small eggplant, chopped

1 medium-sized red bell pepper, chopped

1 cup of sweet potatoes, chopped

2 garlic cloves, crushed

3 tbsp of olive oil

½ tsp of black pepper, ground

1 tsp of salt

Preparation:

Peel the eggplants and chop into small chunks. Place them in a large bowl and generously sprinkle with salt. Set aside for 15 minutes to get rid of the bitterness of the eggplant. Rinse well and pat dry with a kitchen paper. Set aside.

Wash, peel, and chop other vegetables. Rinse well the eggplants and place in a crock pot along with other vegetables. Sprinkle with pepper and pour water enough to cover all ingredients.

Cover with a lid and cook for 2 hours on low temperature, stirring occasionally.

Nutritional information per serving: Kcal: 153, Protein: 2.3g, Carbs: 18.9g, Fats: 8.8g

37.   Marinated Mackerel Fillets

Ingredients:

1 lb of mackerel fillets

4 garlic cloves, crushed

2 tbsp of fresh parsley, finely chopped

½ cup of olive oil

2 tbsp of lemon juice, freshly squeezed

¼ tsp of black pepper, freshly ground

1 tbsp of fresh rosemary, finely chopped

1 tsp of balsamic vinegar

Preparation:

In a large bowl, combine garlic, oil, lemon, pepper, rosemary, and vinegar. Mix well and soak the fillets in this marinade. Cover with a plastic foil and refrigerate for about 30 minutes.

Preheat the grill to a medium-high temperature. Drain the fillets and reserve the marinade. Grill for 4-5 minutes on each side, or until desired doneness.

Serve fish with some steamed or broiled vegetables.

Nutritional information per serving: Kcal: 490, Protein: 36.5g, Carbs: 2.5g, Fats: 36.6g

38.   Green Cream Soup

Ingredients:

1 cup of fresh broccoli, chopped

1 cup of cauliflower, chopped

4 tbsp of fresh parsley, finely chopped

¼ tsp of chili pepper, ground

1 tsp of dried thyme, ground

½ cup of milk, low-fat

Preparation:

Place broccoli and cauliflower in a heavy-bottomed pot. Add enough water to cover all ingredients and bring it to a boil. Cook for 5 minutes, or until tender. Remove from the heat and drain well. Set aside to cool for a while.

Transfer cooked broccoli and cauliflower to a blender. Add ½ cup of water and sprinkle with chili pepper. Process until pureed and transfer to a clean heavy-bottomed pot.

Add 2 cups of water and sprinkle with finely chopped parsley. Bring it to a boil and reduce the heat to low. Cook for 2 minutes. Add milk and give it a good stir. Cook until heated trough.

Serve warm.

Nutritional information per serving: Kcal: 490, Protein: 36.5g, Carbs: 2.5g, Fats: 36.6g

39.   Fresh Mediterranean Salad

Ingredients:

2 large tomatoes, chopped

1 cup of Romaine lettuce, roughly chopped

1 large green bell pepper, sliced

1 small red onion, sliced

1 small cucumber, sliced

1 tbsp of balsamic vinegar

3 tbsp of extra-virgin olive oil

1 tbsp of fresh parsley, finely chopped

1 tsp of Italian seasoning mix

Preparation:

Wash the tomatoes and place them in a large salad bowl. Cut into bite-sized pieces.

Wash the lettuce thoroughly under cold running water and drain. Roughly chop it and add to the bowl.

Wash the green bell pepper and cut in half. Remove the seeds, slice, and add it to the bowl.

Peel the onions and thinly slice. Add it to the bowl and set aside.

Wash the cucumber and cut into thin slices and add it to the bowl.

Now, combine balsamic vinegar, olive oil, parsley, and Italian seasoning mix. Stir well to mix and pour over the salad. Toss gently to coat all the ingredients.

Refrigerate for 15 minutes before serving and enjoy.

Nutritional information per serving: Kcal: 238, Protein: 1.9g, Carbs: 10.7g, Fats: 10.9g

40. Grilled Veal with Avocado and Mushrooms

Ingredients:

1 lb of lean veal, cut into bite-sized pieces

1 cup of cremini mushrooms, chopped

1 cup of avocado, peeled and chopped

1 cup of lamb's lettuce

1 medium-sized tomato, chopped

1 tsp of dried thyme, ground

¼ tsp of black pepper, ground

3 tbsp of olive oil

Preparation:

Wash the meat thoroughly and pat dry with a kitchen paper. Cut into bite-sized pieces and set aside.

Preheat the oil in a large nonstick saucepan over a medium-high temperature. Add meat and sprinkle with some pepper. Cook for about 5 minutes and then add mushrooms. Sprinkle all with thyme and cook for 7-10 more minutes, or until desired doneness. Remove from the heat and set aside.

Now, combine avocado, tomato, and lettuce on a serving plate. Add meat and mushrooms and serve immediately.

Nutritional information per serving: Kcal: 373, Protein: 29.1g, Carbs: 5.7g, Fats: 26.3g

41.   Spinach Carrot Salad

Ingredients:

2 large carrots, sliced

½ cup of fresh spinach, torn

1 large tomato, chopped

2 oz of blueberries

4 tbsp of lemon juice, freshly squeezed

2 tbsp of orange juice, freshly squeezed

¼ tsp of cumin, ground

1 tsp of yellow mustard

Preparation:

In a small bowl, combine lemon juice, orange juice, cumin, and yellow mustard. Stir well to mix and set aside.

In a large salad bowl, combine carrots, spinach, tomato, and blueberries. Stir well once, then drizzle with marinade and then give it a good final stir.

Refrigerate for 10 minutes before serving.

Enjoy!

Nutritional information per serving: Kcal: 81, Protein: 2.3g, Carbs: 17.5g, Fats: 0.7g

42.   Walnut Oatmeal

Ingredients:

1 tbsp of walnuts, roughly chopped

1 cup of oatmeal

1 cup of water

1 tbsp of honey

¼ cup of dates, chopped

½ cup of sour cream, low-fat

Preparation:

Combine water and oatmeal in a small pot over a medium-high temperature. Bring it to a boil and cook for 2 minutes. Remove from the heat and set aside to cool completely.

Combine walnuts, dates, honey, and sour cream in a bowl. Stir in the cooked oatmeal and transfer to serving bowls.

Enjoy!

Nutritional information per serving: Kcal: 397, Protein: 8.7g, Carbs: 55.9g, Fats: 17.1g

43.   Pomegranate Almond Smoothie

Ingredients:

1 medium-sized pomegranate

1 cup of yogurt, low-fat

2 tbsp of lemon juice, freshly squeezed

1 tbsp of honey

1 tbsp of almonds, roughly chopped

Preparation:

Using a sharp knife, cut the top of the pomegranate fruit. Slice down to each of the white membranes inside of the fruit. Pop the seeds into a cup and then transfer to a food processor.

Add yogurt, lemon juice, and honey. Blend until nicely smooth and transfer to serving glasses. Top with almonds and refrigerate for 20 minutes before serving.

Enjoy!

Nutritional information per serving: Kcal: 190, Protein: 8.3g, Carbs: 31.2g, Fats: 3.1g

44.   Chicken Scrambled Eggs

Ingredients:

10 oz of chicken fillets

4 large eggs

1 small red onion, finely chopped

1 medium-sized red bell pepper, chopped

2 tbsp of olive oil

1 tbsp of fresh parsley, finely chopped

1 tsp of dried thyme, ground

Preparation:

In a medium bowl, whisk the eggs, and parsley. Set aside.

Preheat the oil in a large frying pan over a medium-high temperature. Add onions and pepper and cook for 3 minutes, or until vegetables soften. Now, add chicken and cook for 5 minutes, stirring occasionally.

Pour the egg mixture and spread evenly. Cook for about 3-4 minutes, or until eggs are set.

Serve immediately.

Nutritional information per serving: Kcal: 378, Protein: 36.5g, Carbs: 6g, Fats: 23.1g

45.   Beans Spread

Ingredients:

1 lb of kidney beans, pre-cooked

1 cup of sweet corn

2 large tomatoes, diced

4 tbsp of tomato paste

½ tsp of dried oregano, ground

3 tbsp of olive oil

¼ tsp of black pepper, ground

Preparation:

Soak the beans overnight. Rinse and drain well and then place in a deep pot. Add about 6 cups of water and bring it to a boil. Reduce the heat to low and cook for 1 hour. Remove from the heat and drain well. Set aside.

Now, preheat the oil in a large skillet over a medium-high temperature. Add tomatoes, tomato paste and about ½ cup of water. Sprinkle with some pepper and oregano to taste and stir well. Cook for 5 minutes, stirring constantly.

Place the beans in a food processor and add about 2 tablespoons of tomato mixture and 2 tablespoons of water. Blend until well incorporated. Transfer the beans to a skillet with potatoes and stir all well. Add corn and cook for 5 more minutes, stirring constantly.

Remove from the heat and set aside to cool completely. Refrigerate for 30 minutes before serving.

Nutritional information per serving: Kcal: 268, Protein: 14.2g, Carbs: 41.8g, Fats: 6.2g

46.   Sweet Potato with Collard Greens

Ingredients:

1 cup of sweet potato, chopped

1 cup of collard greens, chopped

1 large carrot, sliced

1 small onion, finely chopped

2 garlic cloves, crushed

2 tablespoon of olive oil

Preparation:

Wash the collard thoroughly under cold running water. Roughly chop it and set aside.

Peel the sweet potatoes and cut into bite-sized pieces. Fill the measuring cup and reserve the rest for some other recipe. Now, place the potatoes in a pot of boiling water and cook for 15 minutes, or until tender. Remove from the heat and drain.

Preheat the oil in a large skillet over a medium-high temperature. Add garlic, carrot, and onion and cook for 3 minutes, or until carrot slightly tender. Add potatoes and collard greens and cook for 5 more minutes. Remove from the heat and serve immediately.

Enjoy!

Nutritional information per serving: Kcal: 250, Protein: 3.4g, Carbs: 29.7g, Fats: 14.4g

47.   Marinated Sardines

Ingredients:

1 lb of fresh sardines, cleaned

1 tsp of dried rosemary, minced

1 tbsp of fresh parsley, finely chopped

1 cup of olive oil

2 garlic cloves, crushed

¼ tsp of black pepper, ground

2 tbsp of lemon juice, freshly squeezed

Preparation:

Place the fish in a large colander and wash under cold running water. Pat dry with a kitchen paper and set aside.

In a large bowl, combine oil, parsley, rosemary, garlic, pepper, and lemon juice. Stir well to blend and soak the fish in this marinade. Cover with a lid or wrap the top with plastic foil and refrigerate for 1 hour.

Preheat the grill to a medium-high temperature. Place the fish and grill for about 3-4 minutes on each side, or until desired doneness. Brush the fish with marinade while grilling.

Remove from the grill and serve with some potato salad or steamed vegetables.

Nutritional information per serving: Kcal: 442, Protein: 37.5g, Carbs: 1.3g, Fats: 31.5g

48. Green Casserole

Ingredients:

1 cup of kale, chopped

1 cup of collard greens, chopped

1 large tomato, diced

½ cup of cream cheese, low-fat

½ cup of milk, low-fat

4 large eggs, beaten

1 tsp of dried oregano, ground

1 tbsp of fresh parsley, finely chopped

¼ tsp of red pepper, ground

Preparation:

Preheat the oven to 400°F.

First, line some baking paper over a medium casserole dish and set aside.

Combine collard greens and kale in a colander. Wash thoroughly under cold running water and drain. Chop it and place in a deep pot. Add about 2 cups of water and bring it to a boil. Reduce the heat to low and cook for 5 minutes. Remove from the heat.

Drain and transfer to a casserole dish along with diced tomato. Set aside.

Now, whisk the eggs with milk and cheese in a medium bowl. Sprinkle with oregano, parsley, and pepper and mix with hand electric mixer. Pour the mixture over the vegetables and place it in the oven.

Bake for about 20 minutes, or until desired doneness. Remove from the oven and let it cool for a while before cutting and serving.

Enjoy!

Nutritional information per serving: Kcal: 211, Protein: 10.8g, Carbs: 7.7g, Fats: 15.9g

49.   Ground Beef Steaks

Ingredients:

1 lb of ground lean beef

½ cup of breadcrumbs

2 slices of buckwheat bread

1 small onion, finely chopped

1 medium-sized red bell pepper, finely chopped

2 large eggs

2 tbsp of fresh parsley, finely chopped

¼ tsp of black pepper, ground

Preparation:

Preheat the oven to 375°F. Place some baking paper on a large baking sheet and set aside.

Soak the bread slices in a ½ cup of water for 1 minutes. Squeeze the water with hands and place in large bowl. Add beef, onion, red bell pepper, eggs, parsley, and pepper. Stir well using your hands, squeezing the mixture to get a nice dough.

Spread the breadcrumbs on a large baking sheet. Shape small steaks and roll them in breadcrumbs.

Place the steaks on a prepared baking sheet and place it in the oven. Bake for 30 minutes, or until the desired set. Remove from the oven and serve warm.

Nutritional information per serving: Kcal: 329, Protein: 40.2g, Carbs: 16.3g, Fats: 10.5g

50.   Stewed Greens

Ingredients:

7 oz of kale, chopped

7 oz of collard greens, chopped

7 oz of leeks, chopped

4 garlic cloves, crushed

1 small onion

2 tbsp of olive oil

1 tbsp of balsamic vinegar

¼ tsp of black pepper, ground

Preparation:

Combine kale, collard greens, and leeks in a large colander. Wash thoroughly under cold running water and drain well. Chop it and set aside.

Place all greens in a deep pot. Add water enough to cover all the ingredients and bring it to a boil. Cook for 2 minutes and then remove from the heat. Drain and set aside.

Preheat the oil in a large skillet over a medium-high temperature. Add onions and garlic and stir-fry until translucent. Now, add the greens and drizzle with vinegar. Sprinkle with some pepper to taste and reduce the heat to low. Cook for 4-5 minutes, stirring occasionally. Remove the heat and serve.

Nutritional information per serving: Kcal: 188, Protein: 4.9g, Carbs: 23.6g, Fats: 10g

51.   Red Turkey Fillets

Ingredients:

1 lb of turkey fillets

1 tsp of cayenne pepper, ground

½ tsp of dried thyme

1 cup of chicken broth

2 tbsp of buckwheat flour

2 tbsp of olive oil

1 tsp of balsamic vinegar

Preparation:

Wash the meat under cold running water and pat dry with a kitchen paper. Set aside.

In a large bowl, combine chicken broth, flour, vinegar, cayenne pepper, and thyme. Stir well to combine and set aside.

Preheat the oil in a large skillet over a medium-high temperature. Add garlic and stir-fry for 3 minutes, or until translucent. Add meat and cook for 5 minutes on each side, or until desired doneness. Pour the broth and cook until heated trough.

Remove from the heat and serve immediately.

Nutritional information per serving: Kcal: 277, Protein: 34.9g, Carbs: 3.2g, Fats: 13.2g

52. Sweet Potato Celery Omelet

Ingredients:

1 cup of sweet potatoes, chopped

1 cup of celery, chopped

5 large eggs, beaten

2 tbsp of milk, low-fat

1 tbsp of fresh parsley, finely chopped

1 tsp of vegetable oil

Preparation:

Place the potatoes in a pot of boiling water. Cook for 10 minutes, or until fork-tender. Remove from the heat and drain. Set aside to cool for a while.

In a large bowl, whisk the eggs with milk, and parsley. Mix until well incorporated and set aside.

Meanwhile, preheat the oil in a large frying pan over a medium-high temperature. Add celery and cook for about 3-4 minutes, or until soften. Pour the egg mixture and continue to cook for another 3-4 minutes, or until the eggs are set.

Remove from the heat and fold the omelet in half. Serve immediately.

Nutritional information per serving: Kcal: 202, Protein: 11.8g, Carbs: 16.2g, Fats: 10.2g

53.   Asparagus with Garlic

Ingredients:

1 lb of asparagus, trimmed and chopped

4 garlic cloves, finely chopped

½ cup of sour cream, low-fat

1 tbsp of lemon juice, freshly squeezed

1 tsp of dried thyme, ground

¼ tsp of black pepper, ground

2 tbsp of extra-virgin olive oil

Preparation:

In a medium bowl, combine sour cream, lemon juice, thyme, pepper, and 1 tablespoon of oil. Stir until well incorporated and set aside.

Preheat the remaining oil a large skillet over a medium-high temperature. Add garlic and stir-fry for 2 minutes and then add chopped asparagus. Cook for 3 minutes and pour the sour cream mixture. Cook until heated through and remove from the heat.

Serve warm.

Nutritional information per serving: Kcal: 121, Protein: 4.9g, Carbs: 9.3g, Fats: 8.3g

54. Veal Steaks with Peppers

Ingredients:

1 lb of lean veal steaks

2 tbsp of olive oil

1 tbsp of lemon juice, freshly squeezed

3 garlic cloves, minced

1 tsp of balsamic vinegar

1 large yellow bell pepper, chopped

¼ tsp of black pepper, freshly ground

1 tsp of dried thyme, ground

Preparation:

Wash the steaks under cold running water and pat dry with a kitchen paper. Set aside.

In a small bowl, combine lemon juice, vinegar, and thyme. Stir until well incorporated

Preheat the oil in a large saucepan over a medium-high temperature. Add steaks and cook for 10 minutes on each side. Pour the dressing and cook for 1 minute more.

Remove from the heat and serve with fresh bell pepper. Enjoy!

Nutritional information per serving: Kcal: 365, Protein: 40.5g, Carbs: 4.5g, Fats: 20g

55.   Strawberry Blueberry Salad

Ingredients:

1 cup of strawberries, chopped

1 cup of blueberries, chopped

1 large banana, sliced

1 large carrot, sliced

2 tbsp of walnuts, roughly chopped

2 tbsp of almonds, roughly chopped

2 tbsp of lemon juice, freshly squeezed

2 tbsp of orange juice, freshly squeezed

Preparation:

Wash the strawberries and blueberries under cold running water using a large colander. Drain and chop the strawberries into bite-sized pieces and set aside.

Wash the carrot and slightly peel. Cut into slices and set aside. Peel the banana and cut into thin slices. Set aside.

In a small bowl, combine lemon juice, orange juice, almonds, and walnuts. Stir and set aside.

Place chopped strawberries, blueberries, carrot, and banana in a large salad bowl. Drizzle with previously made dressing and toss well to coat all the ingredients.

Refrigerate for 15 minutes before serving.

Nutritional information per serving: Kcal: 195, Protein: 3.6g, Carbs: 26.1g, Fats: 5.6g

56.   Stewed Chicken with Cauliflower

Ingredients:

1 lb of chicken breasts, skinless and boneless

1 cup of cauliflower, chopped

½ cup of broccoli, chopped

1 cup of chicken stock

½ cup of tomato paste

2 tbsp of olive oil

3 garlic cloves, minced

½ tsp of turmeric, ground

¼ tsp of black pepper, ground

Preparation:

Wash the meat under cold running water and pat dry with a kitchen paper. Cut into bite-sized pieces and set aside.

Place cauliflower and broccoli in a pot of boiling water. Cook for 10 minutes and then remove from the heat. Drain well and set aside.

Preheat the oil in a heavy-bottomed pot over a medium-high temperature. Add meat and cook for 5-7 minutes, or until golden brown.

Gently stir in the stock and tomato paste. Bring it to a boil and then reduce the heat to low. Add cauliflower and broccoli and sprinkle with some turmeric, and pepper. Continue to cook for 5 more minutes, then remove from the heat.

Serve warm.

Nutritional information per serving: Kcal: 256, Protein: 28.3g, Carbs: 7.6g, Fats: 12.6g

57.   Carrot Cucumber Smoothie

Ingredients:

2 large carrots, chopped

1 large cucumber, chopped

1 large green apple, cut into bite-sized pieces

½ cup of Greek yogurt, low-fat

½ tsp of cinnamon, ground

1 tbsp of almonds, roughly chopped

Preparation:

Wash and peel the carrots and cucumber. Cut into thin slices and set aside.

Wash the apple and remove the core. Cut into bite-sized pieces and set aside.

Now, combine carrots, cucumber, apple, yogurt, cinnamon, and honey in a food processor. Blend until nicely smooth and creamy. Transfer to serving glasses and top with almonds.

Refrigerate for 15 minutes before serving.

Nutritional information per serving: Kcal: 117, Protein: 5.8g, Carbs: 21g, Fats: 2g

58.   Frozen Fruit Bars

Ingredients:

½ cup of blackberries

1 cup of cherries, pitted and chopped

½ cup of raisins

½ cup of rolled oats

1 tbsp of honey

½ cup of coconut oil

2 cups of cream cheese, low-fat

Preparation:

Wash the and prepare the fruit.

In a large bowl, combine all ingredients except honey and mix with an electric mixer. Blend until well incorporated.

Spread the mixture on a large baking sheet. Adjust the thickness of the bars with the depth of your dish.

Freeze for at least 2 hours and then serve.

You can also pour this mixture into cups and stick in the ice cream sticks and enjoy in fruit ice cream!

Nutritional information per serving: Kcal: 314, Protein: 4.4g, Carbs: 15g, Fats: 27.4g

ADDITIONAL TITLES FROM THIS AUTHOR

70 Effective Meal Recipes to Prevent and Solve Being Overweight: Burn Fat Fast by Using Proper Dieting and Smart Nutrition

By Joe Correa CSN

48 Acne Solving Meal Recipes: The Fast and Natural Path to Fixing Your Acne Problems in Less Than 10 Days!

By Joe Correa CSN

41 Alzheimer's Preventing Meal Recipes: Reduce or Eliminate Your Alzheimer's Condition in 30 Days or Less!

By Joe Correa CSN

70 Effective Breast Cancer Meal Recipes: Prevent and Fight Breast Cancer with Smart Nutrition and Powerful Foods

By Joe Correa CSN